Getting Healthy
Through Chiropractic

Dr. John Reizer

Getting Healthy
Through Chiropractic

Dr. John Reizer

Dr. John Reizer

ISBN-13: 978-1530048403
ISBN-10: 1530048400
Published by CreateSpace

Dedication

For Kayla and Melissa

Dr. John Reizer

The History of Chiropractic

The word chiropractic comes from the two Greek words *cheiro* and *praktos* which translated into English means the practice done with the hands. Throughout history, human beings have been experimenting with the art of spinal adjusting. There are many references found in ancient records giving accounts of this type of health methodology, which was used in an effort to promote healing in the sick and elderly.

Evidence of spinal adjusting has been found in documents that date back to ancient civilizations such as those found in China, Egypt, and Greece. This information was passed on in secret writings and eventually found its way to the 19th century where health practitioners discovered the same important connections between the nervous system, spinal integrity, and general health disorders.

Later on, an interest in spinal adjustments developed in many additional areas of the world, including America. Medical doctors began to regularly utilize such techniques on patients.

In 1895, Daniel David Palmer, a magnetic healer residing in Davenport, Iowa who was very knowledgeable in human anatomy and physiology, delivered the first modern day chiropractic adjustment to a deaf janitor named Harvey Lillard. The adjustment became famous as Mr. Lillard regained most of his hearing. At first, Palmer thought that he had accidentally stumbled on a cure for deafness. This, however, he found not to be the case as other patients with deafness did not respond in the same way as Mr. Lillard. Although this was somewhat frustrating, Palmer was not completely discouraged because in his failure to find a cure for deafness, he began to notice other physiological problems begin to improve in patients to whom he was administering chiropractic adjustments.

Palmer began to slowly make the connection that vertebrae which were out of their proper alignment were not causing a specific malady in the body, but instead were interfering with the body's natural abilities to process information from the brain. The brain was sending the proper messages for the body to be healthy. The misalignments in the spinal column were distorting these messages and the chemistry of the body began to make mistakes which eventually caused a decline in the health of that person. Palmer rationalized that a correction of these spinal misalignments would restore proper communication between brain and body, thus the biochemistry in the individual would balance out naturally.

Dr. Palmer started his own chiropractic school in Davenport. Later, his son Bartlett Joshua (B.J.) Palmer would take over the school and would oversee the formation of the Palmer College of Chiropractic. B.J. Palmer would go on to perform extensive research in the field of chiropractic and would later author numerous articles and books about the science of chiropractic. He was also the chiropractor who developed many of the spinal analysis and adjusting techniques which are still, for the most part, utilized today.

Why Do I Need A Chiropractor?

Not very long ago I attended a health fair where I performed chiropractic spinal exams for members of my community. After checking a prospective patient on my portable chiropractic table, the man got up and said to me, "But I feel great doc – why do I need a chiropractor?" I hear this same question over and over again from different laypersons I examine at health screenings. The answer to the man's question is actually very important for readers to understand. Chiropractic has absolutely nothing to do with how patients are feeling and everything to do with how they are functioning.

Traditional chiropractors are doctors who specialize in monitoring the integrity of the spinal column's alignment. Most of the spinal problems that chiropractors work on do not cause pain or discomfort in people. They do, however, cause a loss of general health and well being in all human beings.

Chiropractic is often misunderstood by many people. Quite a few laypersons mistakenly believe that chiropractic is some sort of "new age" therapy for back and neck pain. The idea that chiropractic is nothing more than a "mechanical aspirin" has been promoted over time by organized medicine. The origin of such blatant disinformation comes from a plethora of drug companies that relentlessly paint traditional chiropractic's objective as something that is less than scientific.

Tiny misalignments, which can regularly occur within the framework of the human spinal column, can place pressure on spinal nerves that exist in close proximity to the spinal bones. These tiny misalignments, for the most part, do not cause symptomatic discomfort in patients. Spinal misalignments, also known as *vertebral subluxations*, can interfere with the nervous system's ability to function properly. Chiropractors perform regular spinal examinations for patients in an effort to determine where specific *subluxations* are located within the spinal column. Once a *subluxation* is located, the chiropractor uses a manual (by hand) adjustment to correct the bone's alignment in relationship to the other spinal segments above and below it.

Because most of the spinal nerves in the body are not involved with transmitting pain sensations to the brain, it is nearly impossible for patients to determine when or where they might be *subluxated*. Only a skilled chiropractor is capable of determining when a particular patient is *subluxated* and needs to be adjusted.

Sometimes patients will claim that they can tell if *subluxations* are present within their spines. In reality, this is not likely. Patients can often feel muscle pain and other soft tissues that might be injured however, the possibility of a patient identifying the location or existence of a specific *subluxation* is remote at best.

It is my recommendation to the members of any community that every person should get his or her spine checked frequently by a qualified chiropractor. Spinal *subluxations* can cause serious damage to the nervous system and if left intact for an extended period of time, these misalignments can cause permanent dysfunction to nerves that directly influence vital organs and systems within the body. A person's health can decline substantially if *subluxations* in the spinal column are not corrected.

Innate Intelligence

All living things have very unique abilities to be able to adapt to their ever-changing environments. If you think about this for a moment, you will soon realize how amazing life, on our little planet, really is.

Imagine, in your mind's eye, an acorn landing in a field of grass. It becomes naturally embedded in the ground. It receives sunlight and rain and within a short period of time, it becomes a tiny sapling. As the years pass, the sapling will grow larger and eventually will mature into a massive, full grown oak tree that will begin to produce and drop its own acorns. The oak tree is able to survive the toughest elements that are featured in each of the changing seasons. It does all of this, on its own, without a brain. How can this be? The answer is that an acorn and an oak tree both contain an inner wisdom, an inborn intelligence, which allows it to grow and survive in its immediate environment. All living things have this inner wisdom that allows life to flourish. In traditional chiropractic, we refer to this inner wisdom as innate intelligence – the inborn wisdom that exists in all living organisms.

As people, we witness examples of innate intelligence on a regular basis. Think about how we eat and digest our food without consciously paying attention to the complex biochemical processes that are involved in accomplishing this task. The human physiology has to break down the food, absorb and assimilate the nutrients, and prepare the leftovers for elimination. We don't have to sit in a room, after eating a large meal, and attempt to figure out the proper amount of chemicals that are necessary to successfully carryout this very important physiological process.

There are also many other examples of innate intelligence that we can observe on a daily basis. The ability of the human eye to adapt and change its point of focus on a given object, in just a few seconds, so that we are able to perceive the surrounding environment in a very clear and unobstructed manner is accomplished through innate intelligence. We don't have to consciously think about calculating the different distances for various objects we encounter so that we can see things properly. The body inherently accomplishes this and other amazing feats twenty-four hours a day, seven days a week.

The human immune system constantly attempts to keep us healthy by making biochemical adjustments, every few seconds, as we encounter regularly changing conditions in both our internal and external environments.

A viral or bacterial microbe that has, temporarily, imposed its will on a living being is no match for the immune system. The inborn intelligence of the body immediately begins to scan the foreign organism for weaknesses and then launches a plan of attack to disable or destroy the offending invader.

In many situations, bacterial and viral microbes are weakened and disabled through heat. The immune system recognizes this fact and begins to create an environment, a fever, which is conducive for returning the body back to a state of proper health. Very often, people make poor healthcare decisions and attempt to interfere with the innate decisions of human physiology. How many individuals do you know that have taken an aspirin, or another drug, in an attempt to lower a fever or to minimize some other annoying symptom? You probably know quite a few folks that have done this – maybe even you!

Just the other day, I was watching television and viewed a drug commercial about a product that was designed to break up mucus in the airway passages. This drug is an expectorant and it works by thinning out the mucus in the chest and other portions of the body. At first glance, this might seem like a good thing. After all, it produces the desired effect (relief) that a person suffering with congestion might want. But if we truly understood how smart the human body was, we would rarely interfere with what it is trying to accomplish.

In the case of thinning out mucus in our body, we have to first understand that the inborn intelligence in a human being has a good reason for doing the things it does. The body doesn't create thick amounts of copious mucus just for the hell of it. In many situations, the body wants to conceal an active infection or sequester it from other body areas so that it won't spread and do additional damage. After the immune system successfully destroys the threatening infection, it will reduce the thick mucus in the chest and allow the remnants to be coughed up and expelled. Keep in mind, this is allowed only after the infection has been neutralized.

The problem with taking the expectorant is that the product interferes with the immune system and allows the consolidated and sequestered infection to be released through the entire body while it is still active and dangerous. This is not a good thing even though it might temporarily give the person some minor relief from the annoying symptoms associated with congestion and an unproductive cough.

Most symptoms, associated with colds/influenza, and signs of disease are nothing more than intelligent attempts by the immune system to rid the body of harmful invaders. Unfortunately, the educated minds of most people, in society, have been programmed with misinformation when it comes to understanding issues regarding health and wellbeing. A lot of our understanding about health and disease has come directly from giant petrochemical corporations (drug companies) that have a vested interest in keeping you and I sick throughout our entire lives. The products that these companies produce do not cure people from disease. Instead, the products block, in a number of ways, the attempts of the immune system to fight off and cure problems that are challenging our overall health.

Millions of Americans are walking around the planet with a condition known as hypertension (elevated blood pressure). If you ask the average person about hypertension, they'll explain to you that high blood pressure is a disease process. They will tell you this because this is what they have been taught by pharmaceutical companies and doctors that have been taught the same nonsense. This misinformation is repeatedly taught at medical schools, which utilize textbooks that have been written by scientists and employees that work for pharmaceutical companies. We are a society filled with repeaters. We keep repeating the same things over and over again without any understanding of what we are repeating!

Hypertension is not a disease! It is a physiological adaptive process which forces blood to reach areas of the body that are not getting adequate blood supplies. The inborn intelligence of the body automatically elevates blood pressure so that people won't die from a stroke or a heart attack. Strokes and heart attacks are caused from an inadequate amount of blood to the brain or heart. They are not caused from blood pressure being too high. Very often, strokes and heart attacks will occur because the amount of blood, going to the heart and brain, is insufficient despite the body's attempts to raise blood pressure.

The common protocol to treat patients suffering with hypertension is to place the individuals on medications that will prevent the body's inborn intelligence from raising blood pressure. The drugs actually interfere with the nervous system (they disrupt communication between the brain and other portions of the body) so that the blood pressure cannot be elevated even though it really needs to be raised in order to get a sufficient amount of blood to vital organs and body tissues.

Years ago, a *"normal"* systolic blood pressure reading was widely accepted by the medical community as being 100 + your age. In other words, if you were 75 years old you should have had a systolic blood pressure reading of 175. If you were 40 years old you should have had a systolic blood pressure reading of 140. Systolic blood pressure is a measurement of the blood pressure when the heart is beating. The other measurement, the bottom number, is known as diastolic blood pressure and is a measurement of the blood pressure when the heart is relaxed. Under the old system, a person that was 80 years old would be considered to have a *"normal"* blood pressure if they produced a reading of 180/80. By today's standards, the same individual would be classified as hypertensive and be prescribed anti-hypertensive medications.

Most medical organizations today agree that a *"normal"* blood pressure reading should be at 115/75. Anything above this level would be classified as hypertension. How convenient this change, in calculating a *"normal"* blood pressure, has been for the petrochemical corporations. Their profits originating from selling anti-hypertensive medicines have skyrocketed while people's blood pressures have plummeted along with their health.

In all likelihood, the official organizations that conducted the so called *"scientific studies"* that led to the change in how *"normal"* blood pressures are calculated were, most likely, heavily influenced by the petrochemical corporations. By lowering *"normal blood pressure values"* it instantly placed millions of people into a hypertensive category and suggested they be placed on anti-hypertensive medications for the rest of their lives.

The important point that I want my readers to understand is that all living human beings have an inborn (innate) intelligence that constantly strives to keep them alive and well. This intelligence never sleeps, never take a day off from the job, and will be with them for as long as they are alive.

Your own innate intelligence always knows what's best for your body, at any particular time of the day, and it is always operating through the very important pathway that keeps you healthy – the human nervous system!

Children and Chiropractic

One of the most frequently asked questions by laypersons is whether or not they should bring their children to the chiropractor. All children should be under the care of a qualified chiropractor.

In general, children are much more active than adults and they are constantly being exposed to many physical stresses that can alter proper spinal alignment. Regular chiropractic care is going to help any child maintain the integrity of his or her spinal alignment.

Some of the first spinal misalignments that show up in the human spine often appear very early in a child's life. Some of the most damaging forces children will ever face occur during the actual process that brings them into this world – childbirth. Not so much the process that was designed and activated by nature, but rather the various procedures designed by organized medicine and man's educated mind. The birthing process can be very traumatic for mother and child. In the case of the child, the twisting and pulling on the head and cervical spine creates a very good chance for spinal misalignments (subluxations) to occur and sets the stage for an abundance of health disorders to occur over the entire life of a person.

A child's immune system is regularly being fine tuned to its immediate environment. Because biology and science have demonstrated, through research, that the nervous system plays an integral role in how well the immune system functions, it makes even more sense to bring your children to a qualified chiropractor as early as possible.

Proper spinal alignment will allow the nervous system to function uninhibited and without harmful interference that can be caused by spinal misalignments. Because of this fact it becomes very easy to understand why parents should regularly bring their children to the chiropractor.

Chiropractic Safety

If you listen to some of the misinformation that is delivered through the mainstream media, you might develop the general perception that chiropractic is a dangerous profession. This is not true!

Unfortunately, media campaigns are frequently designed to fool laypersons so that they do not explore the many benefits associated with alternative healthcare philosophies.

Regarding this subject matter, reality is often different than what most people perceive it to be. According to insurance actuaries *(people that calculate the level of risk in an insurance policy)*, the practice of traditional chiropractic is one of the safest healthcare professions in the world. Many doctors of chiropractic pay only a few hundred dollars a year to secure their professional liability policies. On the other side of the coin, many medical healthcare practitioners pay hundreds of thousands of dollars during the course of a single year just so they can have liability coverage.

Many medically backed agencies have disingenuously posed as consumer watch groups. These agencies have repeatedly painted the chiropractic adjustment as a dangerous procedure. Considering that within the last fifty years only a minimal number of patient injuries have been attributed to chiropractic procedures and that insurance premiums for chiropractic liability policies are the lowest of any primary healthcare providers, it is almost laughable that organized medicine is able to continuously suggest that chiropractic is a direct threat to the safety of the American healthcare consumer.

In August of 1987, the American Medical Association, the American College of Radiologists, and the American College of Surgeons were all found guilty of conspiring to eliminate the profession of chiropractic by Federal Judge Susan Getzendanner of the United States District court. *(Wilk et al v. AMA et al, No. 90-542 a record of public information)* Because traditional medicine, with the help of other organizations, attempted to destroy another competitive healthcare profession, a high level of skepticism should be used by laypersons when reading anti-chiropractic literature that almost always originates from traditional medical sources.

Strangely enough, most people were never made aware of the fact that there was a conspiracy against chiropractic and that organized medicine was responsible for designing the entire plot. It is the common belief of many chiropractors that very heavily funded anti-chiropractic campaigns are still being implemented today, behind the scenes, by organized medicine and the pharmaceutical industry.

Chiropractic versus Medicine

Traditional chiropractic and medicine have different professional objectives. The profession of chiropractic has the goal of maintaining a person's health by correcting spinal misalignments that interfere with the proper function of the human nervous system.

The profession of medicine attempts to cure various diseases that are affecting the body by prescribing certain medications that reverse or oppose physiological processes occurring in the body and also through the application of surgical procedures which attempt to remove or repair compromised human tissues.

Traditional chiropractic has a vitalistic philosophy which adheres to the premise that health comes from within the body or from the inside out. This philosophy acknowledges the fact that all human beings have inherent abilities to maintain their own healthy existence and that a disruption of health is caused internally. Traditional chiropractic states that if health is lost from within the body it must logically be restored from the inside out.

Medicine has a different philosophy and it claims that the human body is weak and must constantly have its health maintained from the outside in. According to modern medicine, a human being must have an assortment of vaccines and other preventive medicinal compounds in order to build up the immune system.

In summary, traditional chiropractic works with the controlling laws of nature and physiology while organized medicine (allopathy) attempts to go against the controlling laws of nature and physiology.

A Typical Chiropractic Visit

The typical office visit to a traditional chiropractor usually takes less than ten minutes out of your busy day. Upon entering the office, a patient is directed to the exam/adjusting room. The patient will be asked to lie down on a slender looking adjusting table. The patient may or may not be gowned, depending on the preference of the practitioner.

The chiropractor will examine and palpate, (lightly touch) with his fingers, the different regions of the patient's spinal column. The spinal column consists of 26 vertebral segments. There are seven cervical vertebrae that make up the area known as the neck; twelve thoracic vertebrae make up the mid back; five lumbar vertebrae create the lower back and there are two bones, the sacrum and coccyx, which form the end of the spinal column. The chiropractor will also examine the two iliac bones, comparing their alignment in relationship to the sacrum, the posterior (back) wall of the pelvis.

Once the chiropractor assesses the alignment of the entire spinal column, he or she will make a chiropractic adjustment (if necessary) to any spinal segments that are subluxated (misaligned from other spinal vertebrae).

Spinal adjustments are usually made by hand or through the use of an adjusting instrument that has a long metal shaft with a small rubber tip on its end. The instrument is usually able to create a quick pulse or thrust of energy that can be directed, very specifically, onto a vertebral segment. The same principle is utilized when a manual (by hand) adjustment is made. During a manual spinal adjustment, the chiropractor will place his hands on a specific vertebral segment and will make a quick thrust into the patient's spine. Once the adjustment is made, and the vertebral segment has been restored to its proper alignment, the chiropractor will palpate the spinal column again to compare the relationship of other vertebrae to one another.

Chiropractic patients are sometimes examined with analytical instruments that will help practitioners to determine if subluxations are present in the spinal column. Most of these tools utilize technologies that can measure the heat differentials on both sides of the vertebral column. By comparing temperature readings, in different sections of the spine, chiropractors can calculate what misalignments might be contributing interference to the nervous system.

In certain situations, chiropractors will also utilize spinal radiographs (x-rays) to help assess the alignment of a patient's spine.

During a patient's first visit with a practitioner, a case history is filled out by the patient and reviewed by the chiropractor. A thorough spinal examination is then performed by the chiropractor. After reviewing the results of the examination, the practitioner will decide whether or not to x-ray the patient. Once all exam results have been reviewed, the chiropractor will explain the recommended plan of care that will help the patient to achieve the best chiropractic results.

Frequency of Care

It is a common practice for most people to visit a healthcare professional when they become sick. In reality, most healthcare professionals are actually sickness care specialists and not healthcare professionals because they do not see their patients when they are healthy. Allopathic/medical practitioners specialize in treating people who are suffering from ailments and not individuals that are looking to maintain a state of optimal health.

Doctors of chiropractic are true healthcare specialists because they routinely see their patients when they are feeling good and not exhibiting symptoms or active disease processes. One of the most difficult concepts for laypersons to grasp is the fact that many chiropractic patients regularly visit chiropractors when they are feeling absolutely fine.

Subluxations (spinal misalignments) that often occur in the human spine, for the most part, do not cause noticeable symptoms or discomfort. Patients cannot always tell if they have one or more subluxated vertebrae in their spines unless they get checked by a qualified chiropractor.

The frequency of chiropractic care is different for each patient. Every person's spine is unique and so therefore it is not practical to make a general recommendation about how often someone should see his or her chiropractor. Usually, the frequency of visits for a chiropractic program is determined by how long a patient is able to maintain adequate spinal alignment. Depending on muscle imbalances within the patient's spinal column, degenerative changes to the vertebrae and of course a lot of other factors, the frequency of care could vary between a couple of visits per week to a couple of visits every few months.

The frequency of care is always based on objective chiropractic findings that are derived from analytical protocols that have been designed to measure the integrity of spinal alignment. The traditional chiropractor never determines the frequency of chiropractic care based on the presence or absence of symptoms that patients may or may not be reporting.

Dr. John Reizer

Is Chiropractic Addictive?

Laypersons commonly believe the misconception that traditional chiropractic is habit forming. People tend to think of all healthcare professions in the same way. Within the profession of medicine, there are obviously many pharmaceutical products that are utilized when treating various diseases. Many of these products are dangerous chemicals that are habit forming. Because these chemicals are quite dangerous, drug treatments often require constant supervision by medical specialists.

Chiropractic is a drugless healthcare profession and unlike many traditional medical procedures, there is absolutely nothing addictive about chiropractic care. Patients that visit chiropractors, to get their spines checked for vertebral subluxations, often choose to maintain a long term professional relationship with their doctors. Chiropractic is a preventive healthcare practice and when patients learn about the many benefits that are associated

36

with being under the care of a chiropractor, it is not uncommon for these individuals to maintain a regular program of lifetime care.

A patient's decision to routinely remain under chiropractic care is often perceived by others in the community as something that is addictive. Hence, the stereotypical habit forming label is often unfairly placed on the chiropractic profession.

Neck and Back Pain

Neck and back pain as well as many other symptomatic conditions that can make the life of a patient less comfortable are not the professional focal points for traditional chiropractors. Traditional chiropractic has only one objective which is to locate, analyze and correct vertebral subluxations in a person's spinal column. The rationale for doing this is simply explained by reiterating the fact that a subluxation can create a type of interference within a person's nervous system which can impede that individual's overall health.

Regardless of whether or not patients have specific conditions challenging them, they are always better off without the presence of vertebral subluxations in their spines. Subluxations are capable of inhibiting the full expression of health in any individual. Many traditional healthcare objectives focus exclusively on treating specific conditions/symptoms that afflict members of society.

Traditional chiropractic recognizes the inherent recuperative abilities of living beings and works in harmony with those healing capabilities. While it is true that patients occasionally report to their doctors that symptoms are alleviated after starting a program of chiropractic care, it is important laypersons understand that conditions of sickness and disease have many causes that are not directly attributable to vertebral subluxations.

Traditional chiropractic does not attempt to deliver individual cures for specific ailments but instead looks to remove a type of interference, from the nervous system, which inhibits the body's inborn ability to maintain its own health naturally.

The problem with thinking of chiropractic care as a *"mechanical aspirin"* is that many spinal subluxations do not produce pain or other noticeable symptoms. There are many instances where patients are subluxated and not aware of what is taking place inside their bodies.

In my professional opinion, there has never been a situation where a person directly benefited from the presence of vertebral subluxations in his or her spinal column. The vertebral subluxation, always and without exception, presents a challenge for the human body to be able to adapt to its ever changing environment.

Keep in mind that traditional chiropractic can help correct spinal subluxations when detected in a particular patient. On the other hand, the presence or absence of a patient's neck or back pain is considered irrelevant by the focused, traditional chiropractor.

Pregnancy and Chiropractic

When a woman becomes pregnant, it is very common for medical doctors to treat her as if she had a disease. Allopathic practitioners regularly attach a diagnosis code in the patient's chart and proceed to treat the condition of pregnancy as a sickness. Insurance products often cover the condition of pregnancy and so there are naturally many procedures and medical protocols routinely billed to a patient over a nine month period of time.

Just about any other animal on our planet is capable of delivering its offspring in a natural environment without a group of medical specialists standing around a birthing table. Some animals routinely birth an entire litter of offspring at the same time without any complications. A horse, cow, giraffe and countless other examples could be cited to demonstrate that the birthing process is not a disease but rather a natural process within nature that has been artificially complicated by traditional medicine when it comes to human beings.

If it makes good sense to get your spine checked for vertebral subluxations when you are not pregnant, it would logically make good sense to get your spine checked when you are pregnant. It is perfectly safe for women to receive chiropractic adjustments while being pregnant.

There are many ways to modify adjusting techniques through the various stages of a woman's pregnancy and women should take full advantage of getting under chiropractic care during this important time in their lives.

Ideally, you always want your body functioning at its full potential. In the case of pregnancy, when a child is forming and growing, it is especially important for a woman's body to be operating as efficiently as possible.

Chiropractic Techniques

There are quite a few different techniques used within the chiropractic profession. Many laypersons often incorrectly assume that there are different techniques designed to address specific conditions. For example, I have been asked over the years, by certain patients, to administer the same adjustment that I had performed on them at a previous visit. These patients believed that a specific technique was responsible for removing their indigestion, sinusitis or other equally annoying conditions.

It's important that patients and laypersons understand that techniques are simply the tools that a chiropractor uses to correct subluxations within their spines. The subluxation is what a chiropractor must focus on finding. Through the application of a carefully selected technique package; the practitioner is able to aid the body in correcting a potentially devastating condition that robs the human physiology of its natural ability to be healthy.

Dr. John Reizer

Some patients present unique anatomical challenges for practitioners. In certain situations, a patient might not be able to turn his head in a certain direction or he might be unable to assume a certain position on the adjusting table. It is therefore necessary for chiropractors to know a wide variety of techniques in order to be able to accommodate the patients that enter the office setting.

Keep in mind that there is not a special technique that chiropractors use to treat certain conditions in the body. There are however, a rather large number of dependable techniques that are very successful in correcting the one and only problem that traditional chiropractors address – the vertebral subluxation!

Traditional Chiropractic

The human brain sends and receives electrical messages to and from all parts of your body. It is essential that these messages arrive at specific locations, inside of you, throughout your entire life in order for you to remain healthy. The messages travel inside the spinal cord and spinal nerves.

The nervous system is like a giant telephone communication network. It transmits electrical messages that directly affect organs, tissues and cells in the body and it can also trigger the release of chemical messages that allow other modes of communication to take place within our physiology. Whether it's electrical or chemical communications, the nervous system is behind the transmission of these messages and your body cannot be healthy if the nervous system is not functioning properly.

The spinal cord is very well protected by the spinal bones and the brain is protected by the skull. Spinal bones (vertebrae) are moveable structures and they allow us a great deal of flexibility when we are moving about.

Because the spinal bones sit on top of one another, they form a long canal of bones where the spinal cord runs through. The spinal nerves that exit off the spinal cord pass between openings that are made on the sides of the spinal bones.

Sometimes spinal bones become misaligned from each other and this causes them to place a slight amount of pressure on the spinal nerves (vertebral subluxations). When this happens, the messages that are being transmitted through the nervous system become distorted and this causes problems to occur in the body's physiology.

Traditional chiropractors will nudge the misaligned spinal bones back into their proper anatomical positions by making gentle, manual (by hand) adjustments. This is not done to treat specific conditions of sickness or disease, but rather to correct the misaligned (subluxated) spinal bones. The spinal adjustments help to remove nerve interference and this ultimately allows health to be restored in the body naturally. Many conditions of sickness are then reversed by the body's own inborn recuperative abilities.

Afterword

As people, we make choices in life that directly or indirectly affect our abilities to remain healthy. In other words, our physiology is continuously challenged by the foods, poisons and environmental conditions we encounter.

The physiological construct of any living organism is quite complex. Obviously, some organisms are more complex in their design than others. Regardless of the complexity of various forms of life, it's important to realize that all living things share a commonality of innate intelligence. All living organisms have an inner wisdom that strives to maintain their existence in our world. Without this innate logic, living organisms would not be capable of surviving for very long.

In human beings, the inborn intelligence I write about is constantly expressed in the body through the nervous system. This vital lifeline is the conduit that allows or disallows health to be present throughout our lives.

It is my belief that chiropractic is a very safe and affordable vehicle for healthcare consumers to utilize in an effort to achieve and maintain a better expression of health during the course of their lives.

I hope that you have enjoyed reading this material as much as I have enjoyed writing it. The explanations I have offered about how traditional chiropractic works need to be read by everyone that has a desire to be healthy.

Throughout this book, I have attempted to provide readers with pertinent information, analogies and general knowledge about health that I have acquired throughout my professional career as a practicing chiropractor. I genuinely hope that my writings will help persuade people to consider visiting a chiropractor for wellness based care in the near future.

-Dr. John Reizer

Disclaimer

The health information that has been written in this book is not intended to replace a professional relationship between a patient and a health care specialist nor is it intended as medical advice. Readers are encouraged to make health care decisions based upon their own independent research!